Contents

Ramadan Diet

The holy month of Ramadan is the ninth month of the Islamic calendar and a time when many Muslims across the world fast during daylight hours for 29-30 days. The Islamic calendar is lunar and so Ramadan falls at a slightly earlier time in the year each year.

Muslims taking part in Ramadan do not eat or drink anything during daylight hours, eating one meal (the 'sahoor' or 'sehri') just before dawn and another (the 'iftar') after sunset. The end of Ramadan is marked by 'Eid-ul-Fitr', the Festival of the Breaking of the Fast. A special celebratory meal is eaten during the festival, the first daytime meal for a month.

For those who celebrate the month this may mean planning differently for foods and drinks to prepare as well as possibly taking part in online events to meet family, friends and the wider community. Ramadan is a time where it is very important to try to help others. Although doing this face to face isn't possible, supporting those in need in other ways, such as donating to charities online, is still an key part of the month.

While fasting is obligatory for all healthy muslims (not children), there are exemptions for those who are ill or who's health could be affected by fasting, for example, pregnant or breastfeeding women and people with diabetes (see below).

How does fasting affect the body?

During fasting hours when no food or drink is consumed, the body uses its stores of carbohydrate (stored in the liver and muscles) and fat to provide energy once all the calories from the foods consumed during the night have been used up. The body cannot store water and so the kidneys conserve as much water as possible by reducing the amount lost in urine. However, the body cannot avoid losing some water when you go to the toilet, through your skin and when you breathe and when you sweat if it is warm.

Depending on the weather and the length of the fast, most people who fast during Ramadan will experience mild dehydration, which may cause headaches, tiredness and difficulty concentrating. However, studies have suggested that this is not harmful to health, provided that enough fluids are consumed after breaking the fast to replace those lost during the day. However, if you are unable to stand up due to dizziness, or you are disoriented, you should urgently drink regular, moderate quantities of water – ideally with sugar and salt – a sugary drink or rehydration solution. If you faint due to dehydration, your legs should be raised above your head by others, and when you awake, you should urgently rehydrate as outlined above.

For those who would normally consume caffeinated drinks such as tea and coffee during the day, the lack of caffeine during the fast may initially lead to headaches and tiredness. This may ease over the course of Ramadan as the body adjusts to going without caffeine during the day.

Once the fast is broken, the body can rehydrate and gain energy from the foods and drinks consumed. Having not eaten for a long period, you may find it helpful to eat slowly when breaking the fast and to start with plenty of fluids and low-fat, fluid-rich foods (see suggestions below).

Drinking plenty of fluids, as well as consuming fluid-rich foods, such as fruit, vegetables, yogurt, soups and stews, is very important to replace fluids lost during the day and to start the next day of fasting well hydrated. Salt stimulates thirst and so it's a good idea to avoid consuming a lot of salty foods. The pre-dawn meal, sahoor, provides fluids and energy for the day of fasting ahead, so making healthy choices can help you to cope better with the fast (see suggestions below).

While iftar meals are often a time for celebration, with families and friends coming together to break their fasts, it's important not to go overboard when eating during Ramadan. Consuming a lot of deep fried, creamy and sweet foods may actually cause you to gain weight during Ramadan. Ramadan can be a good time to make changes to improve the balance of your diet that you can sustain in the longer term.

The changes to eating habits and lack of fluids during the day may cause constipation for some people. When you can eat and drink, consuming plenty of high fibre foods, such as wholegrains, high fibre cereals, bran, fruit and vegetables, beans, lentils, dried fruit and nuts alongside plenty of fluids may help to ease constipation as well as doing some light physical activity, such as going for a walk after iftar.

Prioritize ibadah, not cooking

Many people view Ramadan as a month to prepare the best meals, since not eating all day should be rewarded with exceptional evening meals. However, Ramadan is an annual opportunity to wipe away our sins, change our life styles and get closer to Allah , so when it is over we stay on the right track and continue the good deeds and habits we developed during Ramadan.

Whether it is Ramadan or not, my food concerns are the same. We fast for the sake of Allah ﷻ, so personally it is not important for me to reward myself with excess hours in the kitchen, when my true rewards are already written down with Allah ﷻ. Therefore, since I primarily focus on enhancing myself spiritually, my food consumption is the same as any other day throughout the year.

Ramadan fasting tips

Fasting during Ramadan carries a high risk of dehydration as food and drink are limited to before sunrise and after sunset. Furthermore, as fasting individuals are encouraged to wake up very early to have their Suhoor (or pre-dawn meal), sleep deprivation and dehydration can lead to headaches.

Here are some tips on healthy fasting:

1. Don't skip Suhoor (pre-dawn meal)

As the saying goes, 'breakfast is the most important meal of the day'. And during Ramadan, it becomes even more important!

Although skipping Suhoor to have uninterrupted sleep may sound appealing, you shouldn't.

Skipping Suhoor prolongs the fasting period as your body will need to rely on the previous meal to provide you with all the nutrients and energy until Iftar (break fast). Due to the longer hours of fasting, you are more likely to feel dehydrated and tired during the day. Furthermore, skipping Suhoor also encourages overeating during Iftar, which can cause unhealthy weight gain.

2. Don't overeat during Iftar (break fast)

Just as it is not advisable to skip Suhoor, overeating when it is time to break the fast can harm your body.

Iftar should be a well-balanced, nutritious meal and not a feast! Overeating and excessive consumption of high-fat foods in particular may result in indigestion and weight gain. Slow down and enjoy each mouthful of your food.

3. Avoid eating fried foods, salty foods and high-sugar foods

It is not uncommon for fasting individuals to reward themselves with rich, greasy, fried and sugary dishes come meal time. While these foods make you feel good in the short run, they can make fasting the next day more difficult.

Aside from the unhealthy weight gain, consuming fatty and sugary foods also cause sluggishness and fatigue. In addition, you should limit your intake of salt, especially during Suhoor (pre-dawn meal), as this increases thirst.

Instead, try incorporating foods from all the major food groups including fruit and vegetables, rice and alternatives, as well meat and alternatives. Consuming fibre-rich foods during Ramadan is also ideal as they are digested slower than processed foods so you feel full longer.

4. Drink as much water as possible

Drinking as much water as possible between Iftar (break fast) and Suhoor (pre-dawn meal) reduces your risk of dehydration during fasting.

Make every effort to drink at least 8 glasses of fluids daily before dawn and after sundown. Fluids include juices, milk, beverages and soups but water is the best choice. Ideally, you should also cut down on caffeinated drinks like coffee, tea and colas as these have a diuretic effect and promotes fluid loss.

A well-balanced diet is key to healthy fasting during Ramadan. Read pages 2 and 3 for the ideal foods to eat during Iftar and Suhoor.

How to Lose Weight During Ramadan

Want to lose weight in Ramadan? We are here with some incredible tips which will guide you How to lose weight in Ramadan. Do you want to lose 20 pounds during Ramadan?

Ramadan is just around the corner. The sacred buzzes of Ramadan arrival are everywhere around us. Ramadan is the month that teaches self-restraint. So, let's use this month to restrain our bad eating habits and to adopt a healthy eating routine.

Ramadan iftar feasts are the biggest chance of overeating and consumption of unhygienic diet. However, it depends upon us how we use this holy month to attain great benefits of fasting by making good decisions about food while focusing our mind on the spiritual purification.

Skip the deep-fried, backed and oily dishes from Ramadan Menu

In many countries, its trend to fill the tables up with lots of delicious food including deep-fried snacks, backed food items, grilled and greasy dishes.

It would be good to avoid such food items with some healthy diet. Such as the deep fried snacks like samosa, pakora, and fried chicken can be replaced with fruits. And the best way for the purpose of to refresh the stomach is the usage of fruits. Fruits provide the energy required for the human body to work properly and help in weight loss.

Avoid the use of starches by skipping the use of bread, pasta, high sugar foods, and fruits. Replace processed foods like soda and deserts with alternative sweets that contain fewer calories.

Eat balanced meals

In Ramadan, the iftar meal is the major cause of an unbalanced diet and overeating. It's the common thinking that you have to eat enough food which should make up for the fasting hours that you have spent without food. But that's not the case.

During fasting, the human metabolism slows down and the energy needs of the body decrease as well. Don't think that you have eaten nothing all day, and eat just according to your regular diet plan. Use dates to break the fast as it provides enough energy and sugar which the body requires after a fast. One date is enough for this purpose because dates contain a high amount of sugar. Avoid the creamy dishes and appetizers that are nothing but carbohydrate packs.

Due to long fasting hours, the eating hours are quite short in the upcoming Ramadan. But this not a reason to skip the suhur meal. Skipping the suhur meal will compel you to overeat in the following iftar meal. In Suhur, limit the usage of salt in food to avoid the thirst in the fasting hours. Eat whole-grain bread, eggs or cheese which are a source of protein, and yoghurt. This food combination ensures the existence of a stable amount of glucose in the blood and you don't get hungry during fast.

Stay Active and do some Exercise

Don't lay down after eating suhur and iftar. We know that it's a tough job to walk after iftar but it will help you to burn some calories and keep you active.

If we talk about suhur, it's a common habit to sleep after Namaz-e-Fajar. By doing this we waste the golden chance to do some exercise which could help us to lose weight in Ramadan. Sleeping after suhur meal is common in Pakistan which makes people lazy throughout the day and increases the chances of obesity.

Don't spend your whole day in sleep as an excuse for fasting. Try to maintain your regular activities but don't go in front of sunlight. Spend your time in offering regular prayers and reciting the Quran as it will also help you to stay active.

More water usage in eating hours

After a daylong fast, drinking water becomes the first priority. Overdrinking of water in iftar can disturb your stomach. So, first, break your fast with something else and then drink a single glass of water or juice.

It would be good to consume more amount of water as it is the main key point to lose weight in Ramadan. By doing so, you can evade dehydration in fasting hours and control the consumption of sugar after breaking fast. But you have to be careful while drinking water in your eating hours. So we have a plan for you. The water requirements of a person can be broken down like this:

1. Drink two glass of water in iftar (One right after breaking fast and one after offering the prayer of Maghrib)

2. Four glass of water between the suhur and iftar meal (eat only one glass of water in one hour)

3. Two glass of water during Suhur meal.

This proper use of water will help you to burn fats, clear the waste items out from kidneys, and clean the stomach.

Avoid the usage of caffeine such as coffee, black tea, and soda drinks. However, it would be good to use green tea or herbal tea as an alternative to water as it makes the digestion better.

Avoid Excessive Use of Processed Sugar

The iftar meals are not a single cause of weight gain problem in Ramadan but the excessive use of processed sugar in sweets and drinks is also a major one. It would have amazing results in your Ramadan weight loss program if you avoid the use of processed sugar and replace it with the use of fresh fruits, honey, dried fruits, and molasses.

If you are going to eat ice cream then replace it with natural yoghurt, mix it some healthy fruits and freeze for 15 minutes. If you are a chocolate lover, then go for low carb chocolate snack bars.

Light Exercises During Ramadan

Keeping in mind the amazing benefits of Ramadan and it's spiritual effects on our soul and body, remember to exercise lightly and a bit, to maintain your health. But do not exercise as you did before Ramadan, you have to have a different perspective as well as timings in this month since your eating strategies change with it. If your goal is to burn fat this month, remember to keep a low carbohydrate diet, or a ketogenic diet, that way you can burn your fat on the body easily with less amount of exercise.

1. Before your iftar, walk for 20 minutes. But remember to keep this walk slow and steady, preferably at the rate of 3.0 if you're on a treadmill.

2. After your iftar, drink lots of water in order to cope with the dehydration of the walk you did.

3. You can do yoga, run a little on your treadmill or just do another type of easy cardio after your meal.

4. It's best to go cycling after your suhur. If you drive to your office but it's not far, try using a bicycle, it'll boost your mechanism and freshen up your brain as well before work or even school.

You should follow the right time for gym and exercise during Ramadan. So, this Ramadan aims to break your sugar habits. You can use fruits which is a healthy option but don't use sugar in the juices which can destroy your all hard work.

So, Friends! If you follow these five guidelines in the upcoming Ramadan then it is assured that your weight will reach a suitable point. I hope you would follow these tips properly to enjoy the amazing results.

Tips On the Best Foods To Eat During Ramadan

Abstaining from food and drink during the Holy month has its challenges but also has its rewards. The benefits of fasting are well documented from healthy weightloss to its rejuvenating effect on the digestive system. However, we still need to take the necessary precautions to avoid any health problems that may arise as a result of fasting. Here a 7 tips on the best foods to eat during the Holy Month.

1. Avoid Processed Foods

These are usually filled with unhealthy oils, lots of sodium unnatural preservatives like high-fructose corn syrup, MSG etc. There are halal alternatives you can use instead so get familiar with your local halal store or enquire with your grocery store as to whether the product you are buying is fresh of processed.

2. Avoid White Sugar, White Bread And White Rice

Examples of these include white sugar, white bread and white rice. These are heath sound bites that are bounced around the media but the real reason is that white flour is often stripped off the nutrition that should be in bread. Whole grain breads and organic brown rice are a lot better for your body.

3. Hydrate Your Body

Avoid tea and coffee as these can by dehydrating. Watermelon is a great way to hydrate otherwise smoothies and natural juices with no added sugars will be just fine. Be careful of spices and herbs that leave you thirsty. Having a warm soup is also a good way to hydrate your body.

Dates are a good way of braking the fast and will give you a burst of natural sugars. Drinking lemon water also has a positive impact on the liver and provides vitamin C and hydrates muscles and this will reduce lethargic feelings.

4. Avoid Fried and Sugary Foods

Consider baking foods that you would normally fry. Fried foods are harder to digest because they are heavy in oil especially if you brake your fast with them.

It is good to also avoid sugary foods to avoid any sugar crashes and consider sweeter fruits an alternative to sugary snacks and deserts.

5. Watch Your Carbohydrate Intake

Rice, pasta, potatoes are all staples in the diet of a lot of cultures and some may wonder what is left to eat if you are told to stay away from these however, these are high in carbohydrates, and carbohydrates get converted into sugar and excess. sugar could potentially lead to problems like diabetes. So these should be kept at a minimum and paired with proteins for a more balanced

6. Eat Dates

Dates are high in vitamin A, B6, potassium, iron, magnesium and natural sodium these a nutrients that are depleted when fasting and dates are good for constipation problems which is common during Ramadan because of the lifestyle change.

7. Eat Raw Nuts

Raw nuts contain good fats which help release sugars more slowly making you feel less hungry and therefore less likely to binge.

Ramadan Shopping List

The eve of the holy month of Ramadan is only a few days away, and if you have missed out on stocking up your kitchen with the necessary items, then here's our compilation of the must-have items in your Ramadan shopping list.

So, without further ado, let's get stocking!

MUST-HAVE THINGS ON YOUR RAMADAN SHOPPING LIST

Date palms are an essential part of Ramadan grocery shopping

Ramadan – the most sacred and festive month in the Muslim world – is almost upon us. Similar to previous years, the arrival of the month means multiple trips to markets and grocery stores to shop for the stuff needed for suhoor and iftar.

Unlike previous years, we'd like to help you welcome the blessed month of Ramadan in full spirit and health, so we have put together a list of some healthy items for iftar and suhoor that you must add to your cart when you are moving from aisle to aisle. These include:

• Berries, Dry Fruits, and Nuts

• Brown Rice

• Dates

• Himalayan Salt

• Low-Carb Cooking Oil

• Vegetables and Fruits

Now, let's explore the logic behind adding these items to your list of grocery shopping for Ramadan.

BERRIES, DRY FRUITS, AND NUTS

The first thing to add to your grocery list for Ramadan is berries, dry fruits, and nuts. We recommend adding these because walnuts, almonds, pistachios, and all types of berries are a great source of healthy nutrients. They are also used in a variety of dishes from suhoor to iftar. They also make a healthy snack for those uncontrollable pre-suhoor and post-iftaar cravings. Snacking on nuts and berries will help you feel light during the fast.

BROWN RICE

One of the most essential things to buy before Ramadan is a bag of rice. Besides samosas and other fried food, we really look forward to the dishes that include rice, especially biryani. So, if you use rice excessively during Ramadan, it is best to replace white rice with brown rice.

DATES

The next and most important item on our grocery list for Ramadan is dates. We do not need to explain the benefits and importance of dates to our Muslim readers. Dates are a quintessential part of this month, and we all tend to fill up our fridges with dates and like to give or receive dates as a gift in this month.

They are a good source of vitamins, minerals, and energy that can keep you fresh and active throughout the day. If you do not like eating it raw, you can find many varieties of dates in the market, such as date chocolates, almond filled dates, or snack bars made of date. You can even use dates for a variety of recipes and smoothies.

Do not underestimate the value of dates by looking at their size. They might seem small, but having a few dates can, surprisingly, keep you satisfied for longer than expected. Moreover, these éclair-like fruits are also a good source to satisfy your cravings for something sweet.

HIMALAYAN SALT

Among the many concerns of Ramadan, staying hydrated is our top priority. It might not sound like a big deal, but replacing your table salt with Himalayan salt can make a huge difference. Since it is produced via natural methods without any harmful chemicals and additives, this particular type of salt is best to keep hydrated and active.

On a side note, Himalayan salt also goes well with fruit chaat and lemonade.

LOW-CARB COOKING OIL

Iftars without samosas and other such fried items just feel incomplete. While keeping yourself energised with the right is among the many essential things to do during this holy month, we need to make sure that our health isn't negatively affected, and we stay productive throughout the day.

Eating a balanced portion of nutrients will help you keep fit and hydrated throughout. If you cannot give up on fried items, it is best to replace your regular oil with the one that has low-carb such as olive oil or coconut oil. Since olive oil and coconut oil are costlier than canola in most parts of Pakistan, you should only use it for frying.

VEGETABLES AND FRUITS

We tend to forget about vegetables this month since it is a month full of festivities. Just because it is Ramadan, you shouldn't forget that vegetables and fruits add a much-needed balance to your diet.

So, this was our list of things that you should add to your Ramadan grocery list. We have only mentioned the must-haves to keep our list short.

We know for a fact that Ramadan 2020 is going to be a bit different around the world due to the current global pandemic. So, we will now answer your questions about what is the best time for Ramadan grocery shopping.

RAMADAN SHOPPING TIPS

Pick up healthy and fresh food items

Ramadan brings in a sense of spirituality and gratefulness. It is the time where we meditate and ponder over the blessings that we have been awarded. We take care of the needy and look forward to iftar invitations. This time around, it might not be the same, and we might not be able to attend social gatherings as much as we did before.

That said, we have to adjust to the change and do our best to care for ourselves and others. Here're a few tips to keep in mind before you head out for Ramadan grocery shopping:

• You should opt for stores that are taking online orders for groceries. Take a look at our recently published blog on stores that are delivering groceries at your doorstep in Karachi. That way, you can protect yourself and others around you. It can also make your shopping hassle-free.

• If you must go out, make sure you are following all the protocols of staying safe from the Coronavirus. You can take help from our recently published guide on safe grocery shopping during the virus outbreak.

• When you are going across different aisles, you might end up adding the stuff to your cart that you really do not need but were tempted to buy. Remember to stick to your grocery list and do not buy unnecessary or unhealthy food items that can take a toll on your health and pocket, too. Further, we advise you to either go alone for grocery shopping or take just one person along to help you load and unload the items. Make sure you are not taking along children or elderly people since grocery markets tend to get crowded this time around.

• Do not panic if you look at another person's cart – you might feel like piling up yours too. You never know the reason behind why their cart contains what it does. They might have a bigger family than you, or they might be shopping for their neighbours or other family members. All in all, just stick to your personal plan of buying.

• Before you start preparing your Ramadan shopping list, take a trip to the grocery market, and conduct an in-depth inspection of your pantry, cupboards, and fridge. Look for things that you already have at home, so you do not end up buying more than you need. Try to use the first-bought item rather than bringing a new bag.

• Do not eat too many fried and oily things. Try to cook as many meals at home as possible. This includes fried items. If you must eat from outside, make sure the restaurant is following all the protocols of hygiene.

• Although we do not need to mention this, you should remember that Ramadan is about sharing and caring. So, do not forget the needy in this sacred month. Make sure everyone around you is fed and cared for.

The Food of Ramadan: When and What to Eat

Ramadan (in Arabic: رمضان, Ramadān) is the ninth month in the Islamic calendar. During the whole month, observers of Islam fast from sunrise to sunset. During the fast, no food or drink is consumed, and thoughts must be kept pure. Followers of Islam believe that fasting teaches patience, modesty, and spirituality. Meals are served before sunrise, called suhoor, and after sunset, called iftar, and eaten with family or with the local community.

Who Fasts and Who Doesn't

The fast is strictly observed, even in higher latitudes, by all adult Muslims. The elderly, sick, and mentally ill are exempt from the fasting. Also exempt are pregnant women, women during the period of their menstruation, and women nursing their newborns. In some Muslim communities, people who miss the fasting portion of Ramadan generously feed the poor and unfortunate during the suhoor and iftar meals.

Suhoor and Iftar

During Ramadan, two main meals are served: suhoor, which is served before dawn, and iftar, which is served after sunset. Suhoor should be a hearty, healthy meal to provide needed energy throughout a day of fasting — it ends when the sun rises and the fajr, or morning prayer, begins.

At the end of the day, when the sun sets, the maghrib prayer starts, and the day's fast is broken with iftar. Many Muslims break their fast by eating dates before beginning the iftar meal. Muslims can continue eating and drinking throughout the night until the next day's suhoor. At the end of the Ramadan month, Muslims celebrate the Festival of Fast-Breaking, called Eid al-Fitr.

What to Eat

Both of the suhoor and iftar meals contain fresh fruit, vegetables, halal meats, breads, cheeses, and sweets. "I try to keep my Ramadan very light and full of fiber, proteins, and complex carbs.. The types of food served vary by region, whether you're in the Middle East, Europe, Asia, North America, or beyond. The meals are served either at home with family, in the community mosques, or other designated places within the Muslim community.

"During iftar, a series of snacks are cooked. Some people prefer to have a few snacks and opt for having a complete dinner after. It usually includes spicy vegetable or paneer fritters, spicy fruit chaat, dal, dates, and sometimes fruit custard

Foods to Avoid During Suhur

Avoid eating foods containing refined carbohydrates as they are low in essential nutrients and can make you feel energetic only for 2-4 hours. Salty foods should be avoided too as they can imbalance sodium level in the body. Additionally, do not have caffeinated drinks as they can cause insomnia and restlessness. Also, tea and coffee can make you feel dehydrated and keep you longing for water.

Foods to Eat During Iftar

Potassium containing foods including potato, broccoli, mushroom, peas, spinach etc. are called powerhouses of nutrition. It is advised to eat them after a long day of fasting. They can hydrate you quickly and rejuvenate your body. Also have sufficient fluid. Raw nuts and hydrating veggies are also good options to have.

Foods to Avoid Eating During Iftar

You must avoid drinking processed and carbonated beverages. Additionally, do not consume sugar-rich or fried foods like chocolate, sweets, samosas, dumplings etc.

Health benefits of Ramadan fasting

In the month of Ramadan, the breaking of dawn beckons more than one billion Muslims around the world to observe a rigorous ritual of moral abstinence and fasting. Practised by the rich and poor alike, the fast requires enormous spiritual discipline to forego food and water for around 18 hours a day. It acts as a reminder to empathise with the less fortunate who suffer the pangs of hunger, thus bridging social classes and statuses.

While fasting during this time may be seen as purely religious, health experts claim there are many health benefits to this ritual of denial and abstinence.

1. Weight Loss

Dr Razeen Mahroof, an anaesthetist from Oxford, says that though the spiritual aspect is emphasised more than the health aspect, "it's a great chance to get the physical benefits as well."

In an article in The Washington Post, Tehran diet doctors are said to be using Ramadan to help overweight people achieve their goals. The common practice for most Muslims is to gorge on sweets and fatty foods as soon as the sun set

– but, doctors would encourage a healthy evening meal consisting of soup, fresh bread, dates and goat cheese.

These foods, which are traditionally eaten in the holy month, are without the sweet temptations and sauces, and thus have slimming effects. With their high levels of potassium, magnesium and B vitamins, dates are one of the healthiest fruits that give the desired energy boost. An average serving of dates contains 31 grammes of carbohydrates.

2. Low Blood Sugar

With long hours of food deprivation, our blood sugar tends to go down. According to Dr Mahroof, the body uses up stored glucose for energy when we are fasting. However, people with diabetes should consult their doctors before fasting for long periods, but those with high blood sugar – but no diabetes – will benefit from the process.

3. Lower cholesterol

A team of cardiologists in the United Arab Emirates (UAE) found that people observing Ramadan enjoy a positive effect on their lipid profile, which means a reduction of cholesterol in the blood.

Low cholesterol increases cardiovascular health, which will reduce the risk of heart diseases such as strokes or heart attacks. If Muslims follow a healthy diet even after Ramadan, they should have no problem keeping this lowered cholesterol level.

4. Absorption of more nutrients

Fasting throughout the day can make our metabolism more efficient. Thanks to the combination of fasting and eating late at night which produces an increase in a hormone called adiponectin – thus, allowing our muscles to absorb more nutrients. Various areas of the body will then be able to make use of the nutrients needed to function effectively.

5. Detoxification

Besides spiritual cleansing, fasting allows the body to detoxify the digestive system as we refrain from drinking and eating throughout the day. When the body starts eating into fat reserves to create energy, it will also burn away any harmful toxins that might be present in fat deposits. This returns the body to its blank slate, supporting a consistently healthy lifestyle.

6. Better mental well-being

According to a study by American scientists, the mental focus achieved during Ramadan increases the level of the brain-derived neurotrophic factor, which causes the body to produce more brain cells, thus improving brain function. It promotes clarity of mind and reduces stress, especially when fasting leads to a distinct reduction in the amount of the hormone cortisol, produced by the adrenal gland.

Besides, the body begins to adjust to its new eating and drinking pattern as higher levels of endorphins appear in the blood, hence making us more alert and happier, thus adding a boost to our general well-being.

Keeping tab on potential health risks

While fasting may reap surprisingly great benefits, medical experts caution diabetics of its dangers. "There are 1.6 billion Muslims in the world and 148 million have diabetes. And that number is growing at a faster pace than in non-Muslims," says Osama Hamdy, Medical Director of the Obesity Clinical Program and Director of the Inpatient Program at the Joslin Diabetes Centre, Harvard Medical School.

In presenting his research on Ramadan fasting and diabetes at the American Association of Clinical Endocrinologists (AACE) conference in Austin recently, he says, "The effects of fasting during Ramadan – which requires no food or fluids from sunup to sundown – can include dehydration, hypoglycemia during fasting hours, and hyperglycemia after the big meal at the end of the day.

"Some of the large, end-of-day meals, which may be eaten quickly because of hunger, can be as high as 1500 calories and usually includes sugary desserts specific to Ramadan," he adds.

He suggests that patients do a trial fast three consecutive days before Ramadan to help them and their doctor adjust insulin dosage during fasting.

Though fasting may cause complications such as heartburn, irritability, dehydration and a decline in concentration levels, its benefits outweigh the negative. "You should have a balanced diet, with the right proportion of carbs, fat, and protein," Dr Mahro o f advises.

"The way Muslims approach diet during fasting is similar to the way they should be eating outside of Ramadan anyway."

Evidently, fasting during Ramadan – if done the right way – will not only lead us to a deeper spiritual awareness, but will also pave the way for a healthier lifestyle.

Diabetes and Ramadan: Tips for Fasting

Fasting during Ramadan is not compulsory if you have chronic diseases, or where fasting endangers or is harmful to your life.

Fasting during the month of Ramadan is one of the pillars of Islam and a duty for every Muslim. At Singapore General Hospital, we aim to support you as much as possible in carrying out your religious duty when you have diabetes.

Whilst fasting during Ramadan brings many benefits to diabetes patients (for example weight loss), there are also associated risks.

Before you fast

1. Know that there is no compulsion to fast when you're not healthy

Surah Al Baqarah Verse 184 - 185 provides a clear guide that fasting during Ramadan is not compulsory if you have chronic diseases, or where fasting endangers or is harmful to your life (e.g. if you're on insulin, have renal failure, or are pregnant).

You can make contributions to the poor or needy in lieu of fasting during Ramadan.

2. Make the decision to fast with the doctor treating your diabetes 2 months before Ramadan

It is important to discuss fasting with your doctor up to 2 months before Ramadan as you will need to know:

o How to fast safely

o Whether adjustments to your diabetes medications may need to be made beforehand. Do not self-adjust or stop medications on your own.

3. Have a trial run of fasting before Ramadan

A "trial run" of fasting before Ramadan (i.e. Puasa Sunat) may be done to identify possible problems during fasting for Ramadan. Please discuss this with your doctor.

During your fast

4. Don't skip Sahur (your pre-dawn meal)

You must not skip your Sahur (pre-dawn) meal. Have a well-balanced meal in the morning and take an appropriate amount of insulin for that, taking into consideration that you will not be eating through the day until sunset. Should you miss your Sahur meal, you should not fast.

5. Choose foods with low glycaemic index (GI) to prevent your blood sugar from fluctuating too much.

For example, basmati rice has a lower GI than regular white rice.

6. Drink 8 glasses of sugar-free fluids

Try to drink adequate fluids (choose sugar-free fluids) during Sahur and Iftar (sunset-meal) to replenish fluid loss during the day. Aim for 8 glasses a day.

7. Monitor your blood glucose levels when you are fasting

Self-monitoring of blood glucose during fasting is allowed during Ramadan. In fact, it is necessary for a successful fast.

8. Check for high blood glucose, low blood glucose levels or severe dehydration

You must be able to recognise when you have high blood glucose levels, low blood glucose levels or severe dehydration.

9. Signs you should stop fasting

You MUST terminate your fast immediately if you encounter these problems. Skipped fasting days can be replaced in the future.

Blood glucose levels

o Blood glucose < 4.0 mmol/L during fasting

o Blood glucose > 16 mmol/lL

Signs of hypoglycaemia (low blood glucose)

3. Feelings of tremors

4. Sweating

5. Palpitations

6. Hunger

7. Dizziness

8. Confusion

Symptoms of severe dehydration

9. Dizziness (feeling faint)

10. Confusion

After your fast

10. Break your fast promptly and eat in moderation

Breaking of fasting (berbuka) should not be delayed. When breaking fast, drink plenty of fluids and have a healthy meal. Try not to go overboard when you buka puasa!

Ramadan and pregnancy

If you are a Muslim woman who is pregnant, or is planning to become pregnant, you may be wondering whether you should still fast during Ramadan. Hopefully the responses to the frequently asked questions below will help provide you with the information you need.

Do I have to fast?

Islamic law gives permission for pregnant and breastfeeding women to opt out of fasting if she fears that it will harm her health or the health of her baby.

Missed days of fasting can be made up at a later date, or if this isn't possible, a 'fidyah' can be paid by providing food for someone in poverty for every missed day of fasting. However, some pregnant Muslim women decide to fast during Ramadan. This is a very personal decision and will depend on your own circumstances such as the stage of pregnancy, how you are feeling and if you have experienced any problems so far in your pregnancy. Fasting should be discussed with your midwife or doctor so that you can have a health check, identify any potential complications you may be at risk of when fasting and get their advice on whether fasting is likely to harm you or your baby's health. The time of year Ramadan falls (e.g. during long hot summer days) and work commitments may also affect your decision.

Is fasting during pregnancy safe?

Research is still ongoing in this area and although the evidence is not clear cut, many experts believe it is not a good idea to fast during pregnancy. There is some evidence to suggest that pregnant women who fast during Ramadan may have smaller placentas and/or babies with slightly lower birth weights, compared to women who don't fast. Fasting may also increase the risk of becoming dehydrated, especially if Ramadan falls during the summer, and this may affect the way your kidneys function and the amount of fluid surrounding your baby. However, other studies have not found any differences between babies who are born to mothers who have fasted and those who have not fasted during Ramadan. The impact of fasting during pregnancy may depend on the overall health of the mother, the stage of pregnancy and the time of year Ramadan occurs. More research is needed to fully understand what impact fasting may have on the health and development of the baby and what that may mean for the child's health in later life.

If I decide to fast, is there anything I can do to make it more manageable for me and my baby?

Pregnancy is quite a demanding time for your body in terms of nutrients and fluids it needs. If you are considering taking part in Ramadan during pregnancy, make sure you let your midwife and/or doctor know so that they can offer you some advice and perform any necessary health checks. If you do decide to fast during Ramadan, you may wish to consider fasting on some but not all days of the month e.g. fasting on alternate days or at weekends to try and make it a bit more manageable.

If you are fasting, dehydration is something to watch out for, especially if Ramadan falls during long hot summer days. Feeling thirsty or having dark-coloured urine can be early signs of dehydration, other symptoms may include dizziness, headache, tiredness, dry mouth and passing small amounts of urine infrequently (less than three or four times a day). If you feel dizzy, faint, weak, confused or tired during fasting, even after resting, then you should break your fast with a sweet drink, to replace lost sugar and fluids, and a salty snack, to replace lost salt, or an oral rehydration solution and contact your doctor. To try to reduce the risk of dehydration; stay cool in the shade, don't over-exert yourself, and try to drink plenty of fluids once you have broken your fast and at 'suhoor'. Remember that during pregnancy, the amount of fluid you need may increase by an extra one or two glasses a day. On top of drinking lots of fluids, including foods which have a high water content such as fruits, vegetables, soups, stews and porridge in your 'suhoor' and 'iftar' meals may also help to keep you hydrated. It is also a good idea to avoid consuming too many salty foods, especially first thing in the morning, as this may make you feel even more thirsty.

Make sure you are still taking your supplements (folic acid and vitamin D) and eating a healthy balanced diet during Ramadan so that you are getting all the nutrients you and your baby need. Also try to eat foods which release energy slowly (low glycaemic index foods) such as wholemeal pasta, wholemeal bread, oat and bran based cereals, beans and unsalted nuts, especially at suhoor.

If you have decided to fast during Ramadan and then begin to feel unwell, it is important to contact your midwife or doctor as soon as possible and consider breaking your fast.

Ramadan Meal Plan

Toward the end of Ramadan I can start to feel zapped of both energy and recipe ideas. I tackle this fatigue by revisiting my repertoire of favorite yet easy-to-put-together dishes. For suhoor, I really need quick and satisfying options that won't make me f e e l too full. I try to avoid any processed sugars or oily foods because they'll drag me down later in the day. For iftar, I'm looking for flavorful meals with little preparation time — especially during the weeknights. This meal plan brings all that thinking into one place.

Maybe it'll inspire you as you plan for the coming week of meals.

Sunday

Sunday is the day I use to get ready for the week — Ramadan or not. It's perhaps even more important during this month, since the work day is long and all I usually want is a nap when I get home. My meals have to be quick and easy enough for me to want to prepare them.

Sahoor: These buttermilk pancakes with orange zest aren't your typical fluffy pancakes, but they're still filling. Plus, the orange zest gives them a nice zing.

Iftar: This spread has a surprising blend of flavors that just go so well together. The rack of lamb is incredibly flavorful due to the spices and dates, and the creamy yogurt sauce is great for dipping the lamb into. A light bulgur salad rounds out the meal with something full of veggies and contrasting textures.

· Rack of Lamb with Dates & Moroccan Spices

· Yogurt Sauce

· Easy Vegetable and Bulgur Salad

Monday

Monday means getting back to work and a weekly routine. It also means having to survive the daily grind while still fasting, so meals should be easy and quick enough to get on the table on time. You can also still follow the Meatless Monday trend with these vegetarian dishes.

Sahoor: We always have a plethora of dates in Ramadan, so why not add them to smoothies, with the addition of a fresh seasonal fruit like apricots? This recipe is one of my go-tos.

Iftar: I love the vegetarian Mediterranean flair of this menu because it's hearty but not too filling. The eggs in the frittata provide protein and the salad adds the crunchy texture to go along with it.

· Roasted Red Pepper Frittata

· Mediterranean Salad with Nasturtium Flowers

Tuesday

On Tuesday I might have some leftovers from the previous day's meals but if not, there's no need to worry because this day's meals are quick and easy to throw together. Since the ingredients are all so fresh and seasonal, they're also just delightful to bring together in these dishes.

Sahoor: If you can get your hands on fresh figs, which are usually readily available in the summer, you must try this combination with bananas in this fig and banana smoothie. It has such a wonderful, creamy texture and it's quite filling as an early morning meal before the fasting day.

Iftar: This menu is so light, but it's also refreshing and hydrating because of the coconut water and the watermelon salad. Also, I love a good wrap for iftar, which can be a wonderful break from firing up too many pans on the stove just to make the main m e a l.

· Fruit Flavored Coconut Water

· Chicken Pita Rolls

· Watermelon Feta Salad

Wednesday

I won't let the middle-of-the-week slump get me down with too much cooking on an already busy and difficult day, which is why I like this very light and refreshing summer menu of soup, salad, and a lovely limeade drink to top it all off.

Sahoor: Banana date cups can be wonderful to have at either suhoor or iftar, but in the early morning hours it's easy on the stomach yet has enough substance to keep you satisfied without adding any processed sugars.

Iftar: This is a super-light menu for that middle-of-the-week cooking most of us just really don't want to do at all. I like to keep it vegetarian, but you could certainly add meat like shredded chicken to either the soup or the salad, or both.

· Summer Greens Soup with Orzo

· Open-Faced Strawberry Pita Salads

· Limeade

Thursday

It's so close to the end of the week, but with one more day to go before the weekend I feel as though I just need to pamper myself a bit and have breakfast for iftar. It's super quick and super comforting and if I have any leftovers, it's perfect for the n e xt morning's suhoor, too.

Sahoor: Strawberry, pineapple, mango and spinach may seem like an unlikely combination of ingredients for a smoothie, but they go together so well and make for a delicious drink that really can hold you over for much of the day. Pair it with a nice hot bowl of oatmeal for an even more substantial suhoor.

Iftar: Sometimes I love eggs for dinner, just like other breakfast items. Somehow they're comforting and hearty at the same time, and they make me feel like I'm not really making too much effort to put a three-course meal on the table, but still eating enough to feel satisfied. Eggs with sejouk is hearty and color, thanks to the sejouk, a Turkish-style spiced sausage, is a great substitute for chorizo and goes so well with eggs. If you don't want to actually cook with it, just cut a few pieces up and keep it on the side of the eggs when serving.

Friday

Just making it to Friday makes it worthy of a celebration! I love something fun and festive on Fridays, so I make food that is a little different from the norm but not too labor-intensive.

Sahoor: This green breakfast smoothie has a banana, kale, apple, and an avocado to smooth it out. Feel free to sweet up the greens and fruit to suit your own tastes.

Iftar: I'm a huge fan of all the vegetables and fruits in this menu, making it a healthy and refreshing one. Substitute ground turkey or beef for the chicken in the eggplant and the results will be just as delicious.

· Ground Chicken Stuffed Eggplant

· Strawberry Lemonade

Saturday

A great way to end the week is to make something that will lend itself to other meals, which is totally possible when cooking a large chunk of meat such as a leg of lamb. Make a great salad to go along with it and you'll be eating healthy while feeling fully satisfied, too.

Sahoor: If you want a taste of the tropics, this smoothie is the thing to make. With the perfect combination of pineapple, bananas, and coconut flakes (substitute coconut water if you don't have the flakes), it's one of the best drinks in my recipe box.

Iftar: Once cooked, this lamb can be thinly cut to make into sandwiches for the next iftar meal or cooked further and shredded for the most delicious tacos.

· Oven-Roasted Boneless Leg of Lamb is a great dish to make for a crowd because it will provide a lot of leftovers for the remainder of the weekend. You can serve it in slices with potatoes or rice on the side, or continue to cook it until it shreds easily and then add to tortillas for some amazing tacos.

· Greek Salad

RAMADAN RECIPES

In this part are nourishing iftar and sahoor recipes for you to enjoy while also looking after your health.

Spiced carrot, chickpea & almond pilaf

Preparation time

40 minutes

Ingredients

- 1 tbsp olive oil

- 2 onions , finely chopped

- 3 carrots (about 300g/11oz), coarsely grated

- 2 tbsp harissa

- 300g/ 11oz basmati rice , rinsed

- 700ml/ 1.25 pints vegetable stock , made with 1 stock cube (or equivalent)

- 400g can chickpea , drained and rinsed

- 25g/ 1oz toasted flaked almond

- 200g pot Greek yogurt

Instructions

1. Heat the oil in a lidded casserole dish.

2. Add the onions and cook for 8 mins, until soft.

3. Tip in the carrots, harissa and rice and stir for a couple of mins.

4. Pour over the stock, bring to the boil, then cover with the lid and simmer for 10 mins.

5. Fork through the chickpeas and cook gently for 3-5 mins more, until the grains of rice are tender and all the liquid has been absorbed.

6. Season, turn off the heat, cover and leave to sit for a few mins.

7. Sprinkle the almonds over the rice mixture and serve with a dollop of yogurt.

Baked sea bass with fennel

Preparation time

45 minutes

Ingredients

- 2 small sea bass , scaled and gutted (ask your fishmonger to do this)

- 1 fennel bulb , sliced

- 1 lemon , sliced

- handful basil leaves , roughly torn

- small handful black olives

- 1 tbsp olive oil

Instructions

1. Heat oven to 200C/180C fan/gas 6.

2. Rinse and dry the fish.

3. Season all over, then stuff the cavity with some fennel slices, lemon and basil.

4. Scatter the olives and any leftover fennel, basil and lemon into a roasting tin.

5. Place the sea bass on top.

6. Drizzle each fish with the oil and bake for about 30 mins or until cooked through and starting to brown.

Cinnamon porridge with banana & berries

Preparation time

20 minutes

Ingredients

• 100g porridge oats

• ½ tsp cinnamon , plus extra to serve

• 4 tsp demerara sugar

• 450ml skimmed milk

• 3 bananas , sliced

• 400g punnet strawberries , hulled and halved

• 150g pot fat-free natural yogurt

Instructions

1. In a medium-sized saucepan, mix the oats, cinnamon, sugar, milk and half the sliced bananas.

2. Bring to the boil, stirring occasionally.

3. Turn down the heat and cook for 4-5 mins, stirring all the time.

4. Remove and divide between 4 bowls, top with the remaining banana, strawberries, a dollop of yogurt and a sprinkle of cinnamon.

Sunshine Smoothie

Preparation time

5 minutes

Ingredients

• 500ml carrot juice, chilled

• 200g pineapple (fresh or canned)

- 2 bananas, broken into chunks

- small piece ginger, peeled

- 20g cashew nuts

- juice 1 lime

Instructions

1. Put the ingredients in a blender and whizz until smooth.

2. Drink straight away or pour into a bottle to drink on the go. Will keep in the fridge for a day.

Kedgeree with poached egg

Preparation time

30 minutes

Ingredients

- 300g long grain rice

- 2 tbsp olive oil

- 1 onion , finely chopped

- 2 garlic cloves , finely chopped

- 390g pack fish pie mix, defrosted if frozen

- 1 heaped tbsp mild or medium curry powder

- juice 1 lemon

- ¼ small pack parsley , chopped

- 4 eggs

Instructions

1. Cook the rice following pack instructions, then drain and set aside.

2. Meanwhile, heat 1 tbsp of the oil in a non-stick frying pan and cook the onion and garlic for 5 mins.

3. Toss the fish pieces with the curry powder and remaining oil.

4. Add to the pan. Cook for another 5 mins, stirring carefully and turning the fish.

5. Add the rice to the pan and turn up the heat, then stir well (the fish will break up a little).

6. Cook for 1-2 mins, then stir in the lemon and parsley.

7. Turn the heat down as low as it will go, and put on a lid.

8. Bring a pan of water to the boil, turn down the heat and poach the eggs.

9. Season the kedgeree and divide between plates, topping each with a poached egg.

Pea pakora pockets

Preparation time

40 minutes

Ingredients

- 500g floury potato , cut into chunks

- 200g frozen pea

* 4-5 tsp curry powder (choose your favourite)

* 200ml natural yogurt

* small bunch mint , half roughly chopped

* 6 white or wholemeal pitta breads , halved

* ½ iceberg lettuce , shredded, to serve

* ½ red onion , sliced

Instructions

1. Heat oven to 200C/fan 180C/gas 6.

2. Boil the potatoes for about 8 mins until tender, throwing in the peas for the final few mins.

3. Drain well, pick out the potato, then return to the saucepan with a third of the peas.

4. Add the curry powder and some seasoning, then mash together over a low heat – this will help to dry out the veg.

5. Stir in the remaining peas.

6. Using 2 tablespoons, shape the mix into rough rugby ball shapes (you should get about 16), then place on a baking sheet lined with baking parchment.

7. Bake for 20 mins until golden and crisp around the edges.

Summer porridge

Prepartion time

20 minutes

Ingredients

- 300ml almond milk

- 200g blueberries

- ½ tbsp maple syrup

- 2 tbsp chia seeds

- 100g jumbo oats

- 1 kiwi fruit , cut into slices

- 50g pomegranate seeds

- 2 tsp mixed seeds

Instructions

1. In a blender, blitz the milk, blueberries and maple syrup until the milk turns purple.

2. Put the chia and oats in a mixing bowl, pour in the blueberry milk and stir very well.

3. Leave to soak for 5 mins, stirring occasionally, until the liquid has absorbed, and the oats and chia thicken and swell.

4. Stir again, then divide between two bowls.

5. Arrange the fruit on top, then sprinkle over the mixed seeds. Will keep in the fridge for 1 day.

6. Add the toppings just before serving.

Vegetarian Stuffed Grape Leaves

Preparation time

3 hours 30 minutes

Ingredients

- 1 jar grape leaves about 60-70 in brine

- 2 cups short grain rice

- 1 large tomato finely chopped (about 3/4 cup)

- 1 bunch parsley finely chopped (about 1/2 cup)

- 1 bunch green onions finely chopped (about 1/2 cup)

- ¼ green pepper finely chopped (about 1/4 cup)

- 1 tablespoon minced garlic

- 2 teaspoons crushed red pepper or to taste

- Salt and pepper to taste

- ¾ cup olive oil divided

- 1 large tomato sliced

- ¾ cup lemon juice

Instructions

Prepare Grape Leaves & Stuffing

1. Remove the grape leaves from the jar, and soak them in a large bowl of boiling hot water for a few minutes.

2. Drain the grape leaves in a colander and stack them on a plate.

3. Combine the rice, tomatoes, parsley, green onions, green peppers, garlic and crushed red pepper.

4. Season with salt and pepper and drizzle 1/4 cup of the olive oil over the mixture.

5. Toss well to combine.

Stuff & Wrap Grape Leaves

1. To stuff and roll the grape leaves, lay a grape leaf flat on a cutting board, scoop out a heaping teaspoon of the rice mixture into the center of the grape leaf.

2. Carefully fold in the sides and roll it like you would when making a wrap.

3. Repeat until all the stuffing has been used and place the wrapped grape leaves on a tray while wrapping. It will make about 60 rolls.

Cook the Stuffed Grape Leaves.

1. Line the bottom of a large pot with tomatoes and season with salt/pepper.

2. Neatly arrange the stuffed and rolled grape leaves in rows, alternating directions, to completely cover the circumference of the pot.

3. Make sure to tightly pack them in the pot to prevent them from floating up and unwrapping during cooking.

4. Drizzle each layer with some of the remaining 1/2 cup of olive oil and season with salt and pepper to taste.

5. Place a plate upside down on top of the grape leaves in the pot.

6. Next use something to weigh it down (a second plate works well or a bowl full of water). This will hold down the grape leaves in place, and prevent floating while they are cooking.

7. Add enough water (about 5-6 cups) to completely cover the grape leaves and the plate.

8. Then cover the pot and cook on medium heat for 30 minutes, until most of the water is absorbed and the rice is cooked.

9. Add the lemon juice on top of the grape leaves, then cook on low heat for an additional 45 minutes.

10. Remove from heat and let rest for 30 minutes.

11. Transfer to a dish and enjoy warm or at room temperature.

Lebanese Fattoush Salad

Preparation time

15 minutes

Ingredients

Salad

- 1 large double ply pita bread cut into triangles

- 3 tablespoon olive oil

- Kosher salt to taste

- Freshly cracked pepper to taste

- 1 large head of romaine lettuce chopped

- 1 large vine-ripe tomato diced

- 2-3 Persian cucumbers quartered

- 1/2 a large green pepper chopped

- 5 radishes diced

- 2 green onions/scallions chopped

- 1/4 cup fresh chopped parsley

Dressing

- 3 tablespoon olive oil

- 2 tablespoon lemon juice

- 2 garlic cloves pressed or grated

- 1 teaspoon sumac substitute grated lemon zest

- 1 teaspoon pomegranate molasses substitute balsamic glaze

- 1/2 teaspoon mint fresh or dried

- 1/2 teaspoon kosher salt

- Fresh cracked black pepper to taste

Instructions

1. In a large skillet, heat 3 tablespoons of extra virgin olive oil on medium heat.

2. Add the pita bread and season with kosher salt and freshly cracker peppers.

3. Fry the pita for 5-7 minutes until the pieces are crispy and golden in color. (Alternatively, bake the pita bread at 425F° for 5-10 minutes.)

4. Set the fried bread aside.

5. In a large bowl, add the salad dressing ingredients: olive oil, lemon juice, garlic, sumac, pomegranate molasses, mint, salt and pepper.

6. Whisk together until the dressing is emulsified and well blended.

7. Add the lettuce, tomatoes, cucumbers, green peppers, radishes, green onions and parsley to the large bowl of dressing and toss to combine.

8. Add the fried pita bread to the salad immediately before serving and gently toss again.

9. Serve chilled or at room temperature.

Vegetarian Lemon Rice Soup

Preparation time

40 minutes

Ingredients

- 1 tablespoon olive oil

- 1 large onion chopped

- 2 large carrots halved lengthwise and finely sliced

- 3 celery stalks chopped

- 3 garlic cloves minced

- ½ teaspoon dried oregano

- 32 oz low-sodium vegetable broth

- 4 cups of water

- 1 zucchini small diced

- 1/2 cup short-grain rice

- 1 bay leaf

- 1/8 to 1/4 cup fresh lemon juice

Instructions

1. Heat the olive oil over medium heat.

2. Add the onion, carrots, celery and garlic.

3. Cook for 5 minutes until vegetables are soft.

4. Add the oregano, salt and pepper and stir.

5. Pour the vegetable broth and water and bring to a boil.

6. Stir in the zucchini, rice and bay leaf.

7. Reduce heat to a low simmer and cook covered for 20 minutes until rice is fluffy and cooked through.

8. Reduce heat to low and stir in as much of the lemon juice as you'd like.

Mediterranean White Bean Soup

Preparation time

35 minutes

Instructions

- 1 tablespoon olive oil

- 1 large onion chopped

- 2 garlic cloves minced

- 1 large carrot chopped

- 1 celery rib chopped

- 6 cups vegetable broth

- 1 teaspoon dried thyme

- ½ teaspoon oregano

- 1 teaspoon kosher salt

- ½ teaspoon black pepper

- 3 15-ounces canned white beans drained and rinsed

- 2 cups baby spinach

- Fresh parsley for serving

- Grated parmesan cheese for serving

Instructions

1. In a large pot or saucepan, heat olive over medium high heat.

2. Add onions and cook until onions are translucent, about 3-5 minutes.

3.   Add   the   garlic,   carrots,   celery,   thyme, oregano,   salt   and   pepper,   and   cook   for   an additional 2-3 minutes.

4.   Add vegetable broth and beans, bring to a boil, reduce heat and simmer for 15 minutes to combine all of the flavors together.

5. Stir in the spinach and continue to simmer until the spinach wilts, about 2 minutes

6. Remove from heat, sprinkle fresh parsley and grated parmesan cheese, if desired, and serve immediately

Hummus with Ground Beef

Preparation time

20 minutes

Ingredients

For the Hummus

- 1 15 oz can chickpeas/garbanzo beans

- 3 tablespoons lemon juice

- 2 tablespoons tahini

- 1-2 garlic cloves

- ½ teaspoon salt

For the Ground Beef & Toasted Pine Nuts

- 3 tablespoons pine nuts

- 1 ½ tablespoons extra virgin olive oil divided

- ½ pound lean ground beef

- 1 teaspoon 7 spice seasoning or cinnamon/All Spice

- ½ teaspoon salt

- ¼ teaspoon black pepper

- fresh parsley for serving

- Olive oil for serving

Instructions

For the Hummus

1. Place chickpeas in a bowl of water and rub them together to peel the skin (optional step, but helps create a creamy texture).

2. Drain the garbanzo beans and transfer them to a food processor.

3. Blend them alone until they become powder-like, scraping down the sides as needed.

4. Add the lemon juice, tahini, garlic cloves and salt and 2-3 ice cubes, and blend for about 5 minutes until smooth.

5. Taste and adjust as needed by adding more lemon juice or salt.

6. Spoon the hummus onto a plate or bowl, and spread the hummus with the back of a spoon to create swirls.

For the Ground Beef & Pine Nuts

1. In a medium size pan over medium heat, heat 1/2 tablespoon olive oil.

2. Add the pine nuts and toast until golden brown; set aside.

3. Heat the remaining olive oil in the same skillet.

4. Add the ground beef, season with 7 Spice, salt and pepper and cook until browned, about 5-7 minutes.

Assembly

1. Transfer the ground beef over the hummus on the bowl.

2. Top with the toasted pine nuts.

3. Garnish with fresh parsley and drizzle olive oil around the platter.

4. Serve at room temperature or warmed with pita bread or pita chips.

Zaatar Manakeesh

Preparation time

1 hour 22 minutes

Ingredients

Dough

- 1 tablespoon instant yeast

- 1 cup warm water

- 1 teaspoon salt

- 1 teaspoon granulated sugar

- 3 cups all-purpose flour plus more for shaping

- 2 tablespoons olive oil plus more for coating bowl

- Zaatar Spread

- 1/3 cup zaatar

- 1/4 cup olive oil

Instructions

Make the Dough

1. In a large bowl, activate the yeast in warm water; allow 10 minutes for it to proof.

2. Add the salt, sugar and olive oil to bowl and use a wooden spoon to mix until combined.

3. Wait a few minutes, then add the flour into the wet ingredients and mix with a spoon until the dough becomes shaggy and you're no longer able to mix.

4. Transfer to a floured surface and knead the dough by hand to form a tight ball.

5. Place the dough back into the same oil-coated bowl.

6. Cover with a plastic wrap or towel and set aside at room temperature to rise for 45-60 minutes.

Make the Zaatar Spread

1. Mix the zaatar with olive oil in small bowl until it forms a consistent and spreadable mixture.

2. Assemble and Bake

3. Preheat the oven to 450° F and line a baking sheet with parchment paper.

4. Divide the dough into 6-8 equal parts, depending on how large you'd like them. Use your fingers to spread each piece into a round flat disc, about 1 1/2 inch thickness.

5. Place 1-2 tablespoons of zaatar spread on each dough and use the back of the spoon to spread evenly.

6. Place on the prepared baking sheet.

7. Bake in the preheated oven for 10-12 minutes, until the dough becomes light golden in color and puffs slightly.

8. Enjoy warm with cheese and vegetables, if desired.

Peas and Carrots Stew

Preparation time

40 minutes

Ingredients

• 1 pound chuck beef trimmed and cut into inch cubes

- 2 tablespoons olive oil divided

- 1 teaspoon 7 Spice

- 1 small onion chopped (optional)

- 3 garlic cloves minced

- 1/4 cup fresh cilantro chopped

- 2 15 ounce canned tomato sauce

- 3 tomatoes diced

- 3 cups frozen peas

- 1 cup frozen carrots or 1-2 carrot sticks, chopped

Instructions

1. In a heavy bottomed saute pan over medium-high heat, heat the olive oil, then add the beef, season with 7 Spice, salt and pepper.

2. Sear for 5-7 minutes until the meat is browned on the outside.

3. Remove and set aside, keep any oil and juices in the pan.

4. In the same pot, add the onions, garlic and cilantro cook for about 2-3 minutes until fragrant.

5. Add the tomato sauce and deglaze the pot.

6. Then add fresh tomatoes and 4 cups of boiling water to the pot and bring to a boil.

7. Return the cooked beef to the pot along with peas and carrots.

8.   Lower heat and simmer for 30-45 minutes until sauce thickens.

9. Serve over traditional Arabic rice pilaf and sprinkle fresh cilantro for garnish.

Almond Milk Rice Pudding

Preparation time

32 minutes

Ingredients

- 1 cup short-grain rice

- 3 tablespoons cane sugar

- Pinch of salt

- 6 cups unsweetened almond milk

- 1 teaspoon rose water

- Pomegranate for serving

- Pistachios for serving

- Coconut for serving

- Ground cinnamon for serving

Instructions

1. Rinse the rice under running water until the water runs clear.

2. In a medium saucepan, combine the rinsed rice, cane sugar, salt and 1 cup of the almond milk.

3. Cook over medium low heat, stirring, until the almond milk is absorbed, about 5 minutes.

4. Gradually add 5 more cups of almond milk, 1 cup at a time, stirring and cooking until the texture becomes very thick, about 25-30 minutes. The mixture will start out watery, but the rice will absorb all the liquid until it is thick and creamy.

5. Let cool for 5 minutes, then stir in the rose water.

6. Serve with pistachios, pomegranate, coconut and cinnamon, if desired.

Whipped Coffee

Preparation time

20 minutes

Ingredients

- 2 tablespoons instant coffee

- 2 tablespoons sugar

- 2 tablespoons water

- 16 ounces milk for serving

Instructions

1. Place the instant coffee, sugar and water in a bowl.

2. Use a whisk, hand mixer or frother to combine. It will take about 5-15 minutes depending on the type of whisk you use.

3. Look for a thickened consistency that's much lighter in color.

4. Serve it as a creamy topping over any milk of choice – iced or hot.

Golden Milk Turmeric Latte

Preparation time

2 minutes

Ingredients

- 2 cups almond milk

- 1 shot espresso 2 fluid oz

- 2 tsp honey

- 1 tsp turmeric

- 1/2 tsp cinnamon

- 1/2 tsp ground ginger

- Pinch of cayenne

- Hemp seeds optional

Instructions

1. In a microwave safe mug, heat the almond milk for about 1 minute, or to your desired temperature.

2. Add a fresh shot of espresso or concentrated coffee to the warmed almond milk.

3. Stir in the honey, turmeric, cinnamon, ginger & cayenne and whisk to combine. You can also use a milk frother, and froth for a couple minutes until you reach your desired froth level.

4. Garnish with ground cinnamon and hemp seeds.

5. Enjoy warm!

Date Cookies

Preparation time

30 minutes

Ingredients

- 3 cups all-purpose flour

- 1 tsp baking soda

- 1 tsp kosher salt

- 1 cup butter at room temperature

- 1 cup cane sugar

- ½ cup of packed light brown sugar

- 3 eggs at room temperature

- 1 tsp vanilla

- 1 ½ cups roughly chopped pecans toasted

- 1 ½ cups chopped pitted dates

Instructions

1. Preheat oven to 350ºF. Line baking sheets with parchment paper.

2. In a medium bowl combine the flour, baking soda, and salt.

3. In the bowl of an electric mixer, beat the butter, granulated sugar and brown sugar until well combined, about 2 minutes.

4. Add the eggs one at a time, then add the vanilla.

5. Gradually add the flour mixture.

6. Mix on low speed until the flour is well incorporated.

7. Stir in the pecans and dates.

8. If time permits, cover the dough with plastic and chill for 2 hours or overnight. This allows the cookies to be thicker more chewy.

9. Scoop the chilled dough using a cookie scoop onto the prepared baking sheet, leaving about 2 inches between each cookie. It should make about 48 cookies

10. Bake 8-11 minutes, or until golden brown and cookie is puffed.

11. Cool for 5 minutes before removing to wire racks to cool completely.

Lebanese Homemade Kanafa

Preparation time

40 minutes

Ingredients

For the simple syrup:

- 1 cup granulated sugar

- ¾ cup water

- 1-2 lemon slices

- 1 tablespoon rose water

For the kanafa

- ½ 16 ounce box shredded phyllo dough (kataifi), thawed

- ½ cup whole-milk ricotta cheese

- 2 cups shredded mozzarella cheese

- ¼ cup granulated sugar

- 1 stick butter melted

Instructions

1. Preheat an oven to 375°F. Grease a round 11-inch pan.

2. Make the simple syrup, combine the water, sugar and lemon slices in a small saucepan over medium-high heat.

3.   Bring mixture to a boil, then reduce heat to simmer, stirring occasionally until the sugar is dissolved and the mixture is thickened but still clear colored, about 5-7 minutes.

4. Remove from heat, add the rose water, and set aside to cool.

5. Use a food processor to chop the shredded phyllo dough into smaller pieces.

6. Transfer the phyllo dough into a large mixing bowl.

7. Pour the butter into the bowl.

8. Use your hands to mix the butter with the dough, rubbing handfuls of the dough between your palms.

9. In another large bowl, mix together the ricotta, mozzarella and sugar.

10. Evenly spread the buttered phyllo dough into the prepared pan and firmly press it into the bottom and edges.

11. Spread the cheese mixture onto the dough, leaving the edges around the pan empty.

12. Bake in the preheated oven until the cheese is slightly golden and the edges of dough are brown and bubbly, 20 to 25 minutes.

13. Remove the kanafa from the oven.

14. Place a large platter or baking sheet over the baking dish.

15. Using oven mitts, carefully invert the baking dish onto the platter so the phyllo is on top.

16. Pour the cooled syrup over the kanafa.

17. Cut into pieces and serve while hot.

Chicken Shawarma Salad

Preparation time

40 minutes

Ingredients

Chicken Shawarma

- 6 6 oz boneless skinless chicken breast

- 3 Tbsp olive oil

- 2 Tbsp lemon juice

- 2 Tbsp shawarma seasoning OR

- 1 tsp cumin

- 1 tsp coriander

- 1 tsp salt

- 1 tsp garlic powder

- 1/2 tsp paprika

- 1/2 tsp turmeric

- 1/4 tsp onion powder

- 1/4 tsp AllSpice

- 1/4 tsp cinnamon

- 1/4 tsp black pepper

Salad Bowl

- Romaine lettuce chopped

- Tabbouleh homemade or store-bought

- Red onion sliced

- Roma tomatoes sliced

- Green peppers sliced

- Beet pickled turnips

- Pickled banana peppers

- Hummus homemade or store-bought

- Parsley for garnish

Instructions

1. In a large bowl, prepare the marinade for the chicken shawarma by combining the olive oil, lemon juice, cumin, coriander, salt, garlic

powder, paprika, turmeric, onion powder, All Spice, cinnamon and black pepper.

2. Whisk to combine.

3. Add the chicken to the marinade and toss to combine.

4. Cover and refrigerate for at least 1 hour, or up to 8 hours.

5. Heat a grill pan on medium high, and place the chicken on the grill.

6. Cook for 5 minutes on one side, then turn and cook the other side for 3-4 minutes until the chicken is full cooked and charred to your liking.

7. Slice the chicken and serve it with the salad ingredients of your choice.

8. Top with hummus as the "dressing"

Zaatar Spring Rolls

Preparation time

Ingredients

• 16 oz halloumi cheese or Syrian cheese soft white cheese like Ackawi

• 16 square 7-inch egg roll wrappers (I use Nasoya)

• 1 small bunch mint leaves roughly chopped

• 1/4 cup zaatar

• Small bowl of water for sealing edges

- Olive oil or cooking spray for coating

- Labneh yogurt cheese for serving (optional)

Instructions

1. Preheat the oven to 425°F.

2. Line a baking sheet with parchment paper.

3. Cut the halloumi or other white cheese block into slices about the size of your thumb.

4. Arrange the egg roll wrappers on a dry cutting board or other working surface, and position them at an angle so that the corner of each wrapper is closest to you.

5. Place a slice of the cheese at an angle in the lower third of each spring roll wrapper, and sprinkle with the fresh mint.

6. Dab your fingers in the bowl of water and rub it around the edges.

7. Beginning at the bottom angle closest to you, roll the wrapper up and fold the edges inward along the way.

8. Roll the wrapper shut, adding a dab of extra water if needed. Press lightly to seal the edges together.

9. Place the stuffed eggs rolls seam side down on the prepared baking dish, and repeat with the remaining wrappers until complete.

10. Brush the egg rolls lightly with olive oil or coat them with cooking spray, then sprinkle the zaatar spice.

11. Bake in the preheated oven until they are golden brown and crisped on the outside, about 15 minutes.

12. Serve with labneh yogurt cheese, if desired.

Ful Medames

Preparation time

30 minutes

Ingredients

- 2 14 ounces can fava beans

- 1 15 ounces can chickpeas

- 1 teaspoon cumin

- ½ teaspoon kosher salt

- Sauce for topping

- ½ cup extra virgin olive oil

- ¼ cup lemon juice

- ½ cup chopped parsley

- 4 garlic cloves crushed

- 1 tablespoon chopped jalapenos

- Salt and pepper to taste

Instructions

1. Pour the fava beans and the chickpeas together into a colander to drain.

2. Rinse the beans in cold water.

3. Transfer the rinsed, drained beans to a medium saucepan over medium heat, and add 1 and half cups of cold water.

4. Season with cumin and kosher salt.

5. Bring mixture to a boil.

6. Reduce heat to low and let simmer uncovered for 20 minutes until most of the water is absorbed, smashing occasionally with the back of a wooden spoon to get the desired consistency.

7. Meanwhile, combine all the ingredients for the sauce in a small bowl.

8. When the beans and chickpeas are done cooking, serve the sauce on top or next to the ful medames.

9. You can have stir half the sauce with the bean mixture and serve the other half on the side.

10. Serve with fresh parsley on top along with warm pita, tomatoes and radishes.

Lebanese Mujadara

Preparation time

1 hour 10 minutes

Ingredients

- 2.5 cups green or brown lentils

- 1 cup rice

- 1 teaspoon salt

- 4 tablespoons olive oil divided

- 6 onions 5 chopped, and 1 sliced

- 1 teaspoon ground cumin

Instructions

1. Rinse lentils, strain and place in a large pot with 5 cups of water.

2. Bring mixture to a boil, simmer and cook covered until the lentils are tender but not fully cooked, about 15 minutes. Most of the liquid should be absorbed.

3. Rinse the rice, then transfer to the pot of lentils and season with salt.

4. Add 2 cups water, bring to a boil, then reduce to a simmer and cook covered until the rice is tender, about 18 minutes.

5. Remove the pot from the heat.

6. Allow the rice to rest in the pot for about 5 minutes, without opening the lid, to absorb all the liquid and steam.

7. In a separate large pan, heat two tablespoons of olive oil on medium heat and fry the chopped onions until golden brown, about 10-15 minutes.

8. Transfer on top of the lentils and rice mixture, add cumin and toss to combine.

9. In the same large pan used to cook the onions, heat the remaining olive oil on medium heat and fry the sliced onions until golden brown and caramelized, about 15 minutes.

10.   In the last couple minutes of frying the onions, you can turn up the heat to high to get a crispy texture.

11. Serve the caramelized onions on top of mujadara with yogurt and mint, if desired,

Sfouf (Turmeric Cake)

Preparation time

50 minutes

Ingredients

• 1 ½ cup coarse semolina or fine, or mixture of both

• ½ cup all-purpose or cake flour

- 1 tablespoon turmeric

- 1 ½ teaspoons baking powder

- ½ cup canola oil or other neutral oil

- 1 cup milk

- 1 cup cane sugar

- 1-2 tablespoons tahini to grease the pan can be replaced with oil

- Handful of pine nuts or almonds

Instructions

1. Preheat the oven to 375ºF and grease a 9×9" baking pan with the tahini sesame oil or other oil.

2. Mix the dry ingredients (semolina, flour, turmeric and baking powder) together in a large bowl.

3. Mix the wet ingredients (canola oil, milk and cane sugar) in another small bowl until the sugar is completely dissolved in the mixture.

4. Combine the dry and wet ingredients until batter is smooth and bright yellow.

5. Pour the batter into the prepared pan, and sprinkle the pine nuts all over.

6. Bake in the preheated oven for 30-35 minutes until the pine nuts are golden.

7. Cool on a wire rack and cut into 16 squares or diamond shapes.

Luxury hummus

Preparation time

25 minutes

Ingredients

• 700g chickpeas, drained

• 135ml extra virgin olive oil, plus extra for drizzling

• 2 garlic cloves, roughly chopped

• 1 tbsp tahini

• 1½ lemons, juiced

For the toppings

- ½ tsp smoked paprika

- ½ tsp sumac

- ½ small pack parsley, roughly chopped

- 40g pomegranate seeds

- crudités and warm pittas, to serve

Instructions

1. Blitz ¾ of the chickpeas and 120ml of the oil with the rest of the hummus ingredients and a good amount of seasoning in a food processor.

2. Add a little water if it is too thick.

3. Spoon the hummus into a serving bowl or spread it onto a plate. Can be made up to two days in advance and kept in the fridge.

4. Dry the rest of the chickpeas on kitchen paper as much as possible.

5. Heat the remaining oil in a frying pan over a medium heat.

6. Add the chickpeas and a large pinch of salt, and fry until golden, around 4 mins.

7. Drain on kitchen paper.

8. Drizzle some oil over the hummus, then sprinkle with the spices, parsley and pomegranate seeds.

9. Scatter the fried chickpeas on top and serve with crudités and warm pitta breads.

Thick yogurt & herb dip

Preparation time

1 hour 5 minutes

Ingredients

- 400g Greek yogurt

- 4 spring onions , finely sliced

- 1 tbsp each dill and mint, chopped

- extra-virgin olive oil , for drizzling

Instructions

1. Tip the yogurt into a fine sieve set over a bowl, then leave to drain in the fridge for 1 hr.

2. Discard any liquid that has drained off.

3. Scrape into a mixing bowl, then stir in the onions and most of the herbs.

4. When ready to serve, drizzle with a little extra virgin olive oil and sprinkle with the remaining herbs and a little black pepper.

Strawberry labneh

Preparation time

20 minutes

Ingredients

- 400g natural, thick, full-fat Greek yogurt

- 400g strawberries

- 1 ½ tsp caster sugar

- 2 tsp rosewater

- 3 tbsp good-quality honey

- chopped pistachios , to serve

Instructions

1. Mix the yogurt with a pinch of salt.

2. Line a sieve with muslin and sit over a deep bowl.

3. Spoon in the yogurt and put in the fridge to strain for 4 hrs.

4. Meanwhile, hull and quarter the strawberries, mix them with the sugar and rosewater and leave to macerate.

5. After 4 hrs, turn the labneh out into a clean bowl.

6. Gently fold through the honey.

7. Take ¼ of the strawberries and purée them in a blender, then fold into the labneh, so you have a rippled yogurt.

8. Serve in glass bowls with the rest of the strawberries on top, scatter with pistachios, and serve with the pistachio & coriander seed biscuits on the side.

Okra Stew

Preparation time

40 minutes

Ingredients

1 pound beef tips

3 tablespoons olive oil divided

3 garlic cloves minced

¼ cup fresh cilantro chopped

1 small onion finely chopped

2 14-ounce packages frozen baby okra

1 teaspoon 7 Spice

4 ounce tomato paste

2 vine-riped tomatoes chopped

Instructions

In a heavy bottomed saute pan over medium-high heat, heat 1 tablespoon olive oil, add the beef and cook for 4-5 minutes without touching.

Flip over and cook for an additional 4-5 minutes.

Set the beef aside

In the same pan, add the remaining olive oil along with the garlic, cilantro and onions and cook until soft and fragrant, about 2 minutes.

Add the frozen okra and 7 Spice to the garlic cilantro mixture and stir well, coating the okra with the mixture and breaking up the frozen okra. Cook the okra, stirring occasionally until the okra is fully cooked, about 10 minutes.

Add the tomato paste, fresh cut tomatoes and 4 cups of water to the pan. Then return the beef tips, and mix to incorporate everything together. Lower heat to low and simmer covered for 15 minutes until sauce thickens.

Serve over traditional Arabic rice pilaf and sprinkle fresh cilantro for garnish